A HOLISTIC APPROACH TO ECZEMA AND PSORIASIS

Inspired by the Teachings of Barbara O'Neill

D.M. CLARKE

This book is intended solely to provide helpful and informational content. It is not designed to offer medical advice, and it should not be considered a substitute for consultation with a qualified healthcare professional. Readers are strongly advised to seek guidance from their healthcare provider before implementing any recommendations or strategies outlined in this book.

The author hereby disclaims any and all liability for any potential consequences, whether direct or indirect, personal or otherwise, that may arise from the use, interpretation, or application of any content within this book. This includes but is not limited to damages, losses, or risks that may occur as a result of following any information provided herein.

The content in this book is intended to be accurate and reliable, to the best of the author's knowledge. However, no warranty or guarantee, either expressed or implied, is made concerning the completeness, accuracy, or suitability of the information for any specific purpose.

Readers are strongly encouraged to exercise due diligence and consult with healthcare professionals when making decisions related to their health or any specific medical condition. Furthermore, it is essential to consider individual health history, current medical advice, and personal circumstances when applying any information contained in this book.

By accessing and utilizing this book, readers acknowledge and agree to the terms and conditions outlined in this comprehensive disclaimer.

From my earliest memories, the specter of psoriasis has loomed large. As a child grappling with the painful reality of eczema—an atopic skin condition that left my hands fissured and sore—I knew the biting sting of this ailment all too well. The only respite offered came in the form of steroid medications, a solution that seemed to only exacerbate my condition over time. My struggles intensified when independence led me to a boarding house where financial constraints narrowed my diet to little more than wheat, dairy, and scant vegetables. Amidst mounting stress, my psoriasis flared violently, culminating in a harrowing hospital stay where tests revealed an unexpected culprit: nickel. This pervasive metal, nestled innocuously in everyday items like cutlery and belts, was a catalyst for my skin's distress. The road to recovery was arduous; it demanded a thorough purging of metals from my environment and a complete dietary overhaul.

But this narrative does not end with my own battles. When my cherished first-born son manifested his own skin ordeal, marked by relentless dryness and itch, I was propelled onto a new path—a quest not just for relief but for answers. The conventional remedies, tepid baths, and copious creams offered him no real respite. It was in this fervent search for healing that I discovered the insights of Barbara O'Neill. Her wisdom, rooted in natural healing and holistic wellness, became a beacon that guided us towards a life free from the shackles of psoriasis.

The journey is not devoid of challenges; it is an expedition that demands unwavering resolve, patience, and a willingness to embrace change. Yet, I stand as a testament to the transformative power of perseverance. This book is more than a collection of knowledge—it's a beacon of hope. It is a roadmap to liberation from psoriasis, crafted to empower you to embark on a journey towards a life of health and vitality.

TABLE OF CONTENTS

1. The Physiology Of Skin and Dermatological Challenges... 1

Understanding the Vital Role of Skin 1

Historical Anecdote: The Goldfinger Phenomenon 2

The Excretory and Absorptive Properties of Skin 2

The Epidemic of Dermatological Conditions: Psoriasis and Eczema 3

2. Deciphering Childhood Eczema and Adult Psoriasis 4

The Age-Linked Dermatological Dichotomy 4

Newton's Third Law Applied to Dermatology 4

The Cradle of Conditions: Baby Eczema 5

Maternal Diet and Its Reflection on the Infant 5

A Case Study: Overcoming Eczema 5

The Triumph Over Eczema 6

Conclusion 6

3. The Complex Web of Eczema Triggers 7

Navigating the Diversity of Triggers in Infant Eczema 7

The Role of Environmental Factors 7

Chemicals, Molds, and Genetics: A Triad of Culprits 8

The Innocuous Becomes Suspicious 8

The Crucial Role of Vigilant Observation 8

Prelude to Adult Dermatological Conditions 9

4. A Testament to Holistic Approaches in Pediatric Dermatology 10

    A Health Retreat Revelation 10

    The Pediatrician's Natural Prescription 10

    The Road to Recovery 11

    Managing Symptoms While Seeking the Root Cause 11

    The Interim Solution: Icing the Itch 11

    Conclusion 12

5. Matthew's Journey Through Adult Eczema 13

    The Early Struggles of a Young Man 13

    A Turn for the Worse in Queensland 13

    The Healing Power of a Controlled Diet 14

    The Tasmanian Relief and Subsequent Stress 14

    Embracing the Gut and Psychology Diet 14

    The Transformation and Long-Term Management 15

    Matthew Today: A Balanced Approach 15

    Conclusion 15

6. The Path to Conquering Psoriasis 16

    Identifying Key Factors for Alleviating Psoriasis 16

    Crafting a Strategy for Victory Over Psoriasis 16

    Learning from the Experiences of a Fijian Family 17

    The Symptom Spectrum of Wheat Intolerance 17

    The Role of Sunshine and Sea Water in Healing 17

    The Necessity of Ice for Inflammation 18

    Conclusion 18

7. The Pillars of Dietary Temperance for Skin Health 19

    The Principle of Moderation in Managing Skin Conditions 19

The Rigorous Elimination Phase 19
The Gradual Reintroduction Strategy 20
The Role of Chemicals and Molds 20
Clothing Considerations for Skin Health 20
Thrift Shopping for Natural Fibers 21
Conclusion 21

8. Restorative Lifestyle Choices for Skin Health 22

Embracing Restorative Sleep 22
The Role of Exercise 22
Revising Dietary Habits 23
The Importance of Protein and Fats 23
Supper Considerations 23
Hydration as a Keystone of Health 24
Conclusion 24

9. Hydration and Trust as Cornerstones of Healing 25

The Vitality of Water for Skin Health 25
The Significance of Salt 25
Trust in Divine Power for Stress Management 26
Internal Medicine Through Nutrition 26
Proper Fats for Skin Nourishment 26
Conclusion 27

10. Liver Health and Elimination Pathways in Skin Healing 28

The Liver's Role in Detoxification and Skin Health 28
Dandelion and Milk Thistle for Liver Support 28
Lifestyle Choices and Skin Conditions 29
Elimination Organs in Detoxification 29
Encouraging Colon Health 29

A Case Study in Healing Psoriasis..30

Conclusion 30

11. Fundamentals of Balanced Nutrition: Harnessing Carbohydrates, Proteins, and Fats for Optimal Health.... 31

Carbohydrates:...31

Proteins:..32

Fats:...32

Recipes: Promoting Healthy Skin.. 34

1. Luxury Millet Porridge..35

2. Quinoa & Roasted Vegetable Salad..36

3. Lentil Soup with Kale..37

4. Buckwheat Noodle Stir-Fry..38

5. Chickpea Salad Wrap...39

6. Exotic Rice Pudding..40

7. Vegetarian Chili...41

8. Baked Sweet Potato with Spinach and Macadamia Nuts....42

9. Almond Butter & Banana Smoothie...43

10. Cannellini Bean & Vegetable Stew...44

11. Natural Washing Powder Recipe 46

12. Natural Fabric Softener Recipe...48

13. Natural Toothpaste Recipe..50

14. Soothing Natural Body Butter for Eczema..........................52

Chapter 1

THE PHYSIOLOGY OF SKIN AND DERMATOLOGICAL CHALLENGES

Understanding the Vital Role of Skin

The integumentary system, commonly referred to as the skin, is an extraordinary organ that demands our utmost attention for its multifaceted roles in human physiology. It is not merely a protective sheath but a dynamic structure that participates in vital bodily functions. An essential aspect to appreciate about skin is its respiratory capability. This function is often overlooked, yet it is as critical as the lungs' role in our respiratory system. The skin's permeability allows for gaseous exchange, making it imperative that we do not obstruct its surface.

Historical Anecdote: The Goldfinger Phenomenon

The significance of the skin's respiratory function was dramatically underscored during the filming of the iconic James Bond movie, "Goldfinger." A popular myth suggests that the actress portraying the golden girl was painted in parts—frontal and posterior separately—to avoid covering the entire skin simultaneously, which could lead to asphyxiation. Although debunked, this tale serves as a metaphorical reminder of the necessity for skin to remain unoccluded to sustain its breathing mechanism.

The Excretory and Absorptive Properties of Skin

The skin also operates as a waste management system, expelling toxins through perspiration. This excretory function underscores the need for skin exposure to air and, metaphorically, to 'play'—to engage with natural elements that promote its health. The skin's absorptive capacity further accentuates the importance of vigilance concerning our skin's contact with substances. A striking example is the anecdotal case of a young chemist in her forties who suffered a stroke, attributed to the transdermal absorption of pharmaceuticals compounded with her bare hands. Similarly, a veterinary nurse experienced significant liver issues from habitual contact with medicinal compounds, illustrating the inadvertent percutaneous absorption of chemicals.

The Epidemic of Dermatological Conditions: Psoriasis and Eczema

In the realm of dermatological ailments, psoriasis and eczema stand out as particularly prevalent diseases in contemporary times. These conditions are not only physically discomforting but also carry psychosocial burdens, affecting the quality of life. The pathogenesis of these diseases involves complex immune responses, and while they may be visible on the skin's surface, their implications run deeper, affecting the systemic functions of the body. It is crucial to approach these conditions with a comprehensive treatment strategy that encompasses both topical and systemic therapies.

In conclusion, the skin's capabilities to breathe, excrete and absorb are vital to our health and well-being. As we continue to explore dermatological conditions such as psoriasis and eczema, we are reminded of the delicate balance required to maintain skin health and the importance of mindful interaction with our environment to preserve this remarkable organ's integrity.

Chapter 2

DECIPHERING CHILDHOOD ECZEMA AND ADULT PSORIASIS

The Age-Linked Dermatological Dichotomy

In the intricate world of dermatology, nomenclature is often reflective of the age of onset. Eczema is a term commonly associated with infants and children, a delicate condition marring the softness of their nascent skin. Psoriasis, on the other hand, is frequently diagnosed in adults, emerging in the years beyond adolescence—typically noted in the twenties to forties. This distinction is not merely semantic but hints at the underlying etiological differences influenced by age and development.

Newton's Third Law Applied to Dermatology

Drawing parallels from Newton's third law of motion, which states that every action has an equal and opposite reaction, we can infer that skin conditions like psoriasis and eczema are the body's responses to various internal or external stimuli. In this narrative, we will explore real-life accounts of individuals who have triumphantly battled these conditions, unraveling the causes and solutions that led to their recovery.

The Cradle of Conditions: Baby Eczema

When a baby presents with symptoms akin to psoriasis, it prompts an investigative approach. Dialogues with the mother can unveil dietary triggers, such as an infant's reaction to cow's milk formula. In such cases, a transition to goat's milk formula, which is gentler on the baby's system, is often advised. The prevalence of dairy allergies as a catalyst for skin diseases cannot be overstressed.

Maternal Diet and Its Reflection on the Infant

If the child is breastfed, the mother's consumption of dairy products may be implicated. Furthermore, the consumption of hybridized wheat, a product of agricultural advancements in the 1950s, has been linked to the challenging digestive issues and subsequent allergic responses manifesting as eczema.

A Case Study: Overcoming Eczema

One poignant story involves a mother whose infant struggled with persistent eczema. Guided by the hypothesis of dietary allergens, she modified her diet, eliminating dairy, refined sugars and peanuts — a common allergen. Alternative suggestions such as almond butter and organic soy milk were introduced, along with a temporary cessation of all wheat products.

The Triumph Over Eczema

Persistence was key. Despite initial slow progress, with continued adherence to the dietary changes, the child's eczema began to recede. This transformation was not instantaneous; it took a full two months to see a baby's skin clear of eczema, underscoring the importance of patience and the persistence of allergens' effects even after their elimination from the diet.

Conclusion

These narratives not only provide hope for those suffering from skin conditions but also serve as a testament to the importance of understanding the complex interplay between diet and dermatology. They highlight the possibility of conquering such afflictions with informed strategies, patience and the willingness to explore and commit to lifestyle changes.

Chapter 3

THE COMPLEX WEB OF ECZEMA TRIGGERS

Navigating the Diversity of Triggers in Infant Eczema

In the realm of infant dermatological health, eczema stands as a perplexing condition, its occurrence as variable as the individuals it affects. Not all nursing mothers who consume dairy or wheat will have infants presenting with eczema, suggesting a multifaceted interplay of triggers that contribute to the condition's onset.

The Role of Environmental Factors

A poignant revelation comes from the examination of environmental factors within the household. One infant's onset of eczema coincided with the family's move to a new residence. Upon investigation, the discovery of black mold in the baby's sleeping area—caused by an unnoticed leaking tap—shed light on a potential trigger for the skin condition. In another case, a new home's recent chemical treatment, unbeknown to the family, became a prime suspect when the baby developed eczema after moving in.

Chemicals, Molds, and Genetics: A Triad of Culprits

These instances underscore the potential for chemicals and molds to disrupt infant health. While there is often an inherited predisposition to such conditions, it is the environmental 'trigger' that ultimately 'pulls the trigger' of genetic vulnerability. A crawling baby's proximity to the floor where chemicals may linger heightens their exposure, leading to dermatological reactions such as eczema.

The Innocuous Becomes Suspicious

In the quest for a healthy living environment, families may overlook the potential hazards of seemingly benign elements. A well-intentioned choice of hardwood floors, for instance, could backfire if the lacquer used contains irritants. Thus, it becomes evident that every aspect of an infant's surroundings needs to be scrutinized if eczema develops.

The Crucial Role of Vigilant Observation

The narrative imparts the importance of a vigilant, investigative approach to identify and mitigate the myriad of factors that can influence the manifestation of eczema in infants. As we transition from examining the triggers in infants to exploring the complexities of adult skin conditions, we carry with us the understanding that both genetic predispositions and lifestyle choices play crucial roles in dermatological health.

Prelude to Adult Dermatological Conditions

Before we delve into the intricacies of adult skin conditions, it is paramount to recognize that the groundwork for understanding these ailments lies in the thorough investigation of their triggers, an approach as necessary for adults as it is for infants.

Chapter 4

A TESTAMENT TO HOLISTIC APPROACHES IN PEDIATRIC DERMATOLOGY

A Health Retreat Revelation

At a serene health retreat, a story emerges that resonates with the power of natural remedies and the wisdom of cautious observation. A guest recounts the tale of her grandson's battle with eczema—a condition that brought his mother to seek the expertise of a pediatrician with a reputation for favoring natural treatments over immediate pharmaceutical intervention.

The Pediatrician's Natural Prescription

This pediatrician, attuned to the impact of diet on health, recommended halting the intake of common allergens: wheat, dairy, refined sugar, peanuts and oats. It is heartening to note the increasing recognition among medical professionals of the link between nutrition and skin health.

The Road to Recovery

Echoing the principles outlined earlier in our discussion, the child's recovery spanned approximately two months. This case reinforces the notion that patience and perseverance are pivotal in managing eczema. If no improvement is seen within this timeframe then the search for environmental culprits, such as mold or chemical exposure, should commence in earnest.

Managing Symptoms While Seeking the Root Cause

While the underlying causes of eczema are addressed, managing the discomfort becomes a priority. There are no panaceas for eczema since the origin is internal, but certain topical applications can offer temporary relief. Coconut oil may soothe, and aloe vera can calm the itching. However, the most effective immediate relief reported is the application of ice. This simple remedy can suppress the urge to scratch, preventing further damage to the skin.

The Interim Solution: Icing the Itch

An itch scratched may bring momentary pleasure but often leads to a cycle of increased irritation and potential skin damage. Ice, on the other hand, numbs the itch, sometimes providing relief for hours. Some have found that applying ice three times daily is sufficient to mitigate the discomfort while the body heals from within.

Conclusion

As we close this chapter, we are reminded of the delicate balance between internal conditions and external symptoms. The journey of the guest's grandson is a testament to the efficacy of a holistic approach to pediatric skin health, emphasizing the importance of diet, patience and the judicious use of natural remedies for symptom relief.

Chapter 5

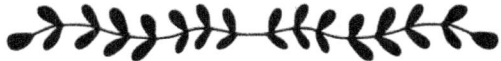

MATTHEW'S JOURNEY THROUGH ADULT ECZEMA

The Early Struggles of a Young Man

Matthew's story begins in his youth, marked by severe eczema that led to contentious debates over treatment between his parents. His mother opposed cortisone creams, while his father supported their use for temporary relief. Despite this, the eczema persisted into Matthew's early adulthood, where he learned that dietary adjustments—specifically reducing dairy and wheat—could manage his condition, although not completely eradicating it.

A Turn for the Worse in Queensland

At 22, Matthew's journey took him to Queensland, where his eczema was manageable until he moved into an old, soon-to-be-demolished house with a mold problem. His diet, heavily reliant on bananas, inadvertently exacerbated his condition due to their high sugar content, coupled with mold exposure. Despite keeping windows open, the eczema flared up, worsened by the hot climate.

The Healing Power of a Controlled Diet

Upon returning to the cooler climate of Victoria, Matthew took a rigorous approach to his diet, cutting out dairy, refined sugar, and reducing fruit intake, which brought his eczema back under control. He discovered he could tolerate oats, unlike wheat, and maintained this diet successfully for many years.

The Tasmanian Relief and Subsequent Stress

In Tasmania, the cold weather further alleviated his eczema. However, stress from his work as an architect and financial strains triggered severe outbreaks. Living in an old student accommodation didn't help, with potential environmental triggers lurking.

Embracing the Gut and Psychology Diet

During this challenging time, Matthew and his family came across Dr. Natasha Campbell McBride's book, "Gut and Psychology," and decided to adopt a vegetarian version of her dietary recommendations. Matthew eliminated all grains and focused on a nutrient-rich, vegetable-based soup diet, avoiding nightshade vegetables known to irritate some individuals with eczema.

The Transformation and Long-Term Management

Committing to this strict diet, along with working outdoors and cutting his hair short to alleviate scalp eczema, Matthew saw a complete remission of his condition. It was a gradual process, taking a couple of months, but the results were profound. He also implemented an anti-fungal diet to further reduce sugar intake, crucial in fighting the yeast overgrowth associated with eczema.

Matthew Today: A Balanced Approach

A decade later, Matthew has reintroduced fruit, a little wheat, and oats into his diet, but the lessons from his journey remain. The careful elimination of specific foods was key to managing his eczema, highlighting the individual nature of dietary triggers and the importance of a tailored approach to treatment.

Conclusion

Matthew's remarkable story illustrates the complex relationship between diet, environment, and eczema. It underscores the necessity of understanding individual triggers and the powerful role of a controlled diet in managing chronic skin conditions. Through patience, experimentation, and dedication, Matthew achieved a quality of life that once seemed unattainable, offering hope and insight for those on a similar path.

Chapter 6

THE PATH TO CONQUERING PSORIASIS

Identifying Key Factors for Alleviating Psoriasis

The journey to overcoming psoriasis can often be complex and individualistic. However, many have found success in eliminating common irritants from their diet. For some, like the individual in this narrative, cutting out wheat, oats, peanuts, dairy, and refined sugar proved insufficient. It was the complete exclusion of all grains, as inspired by a pivotal book, that brought about "total victory" over the condition.

Crafting a Strategy for Victory Over Psoriasis

In light of these experiences, a strategic list can be formulated to combat psoriasis effectively. The foundational step is ensuring the purity of the air one breathes. Mold and chemicals are identified as adversaries in this fight, acting as toxins that can exacerbate or even trigger psoriasis flare-ups.

Learning from the Experiences of a Fijian Family

An anecdote about a Fijian family living in Australia illustrates the variable impact of diet on individuals. While one sibling yawned incessantly after consuming wheat, the other developed eczema. Interestingly, a return to the natural diet of Fiji, devoid of wheat and rich in cassava and taro, led to the resolution of the eczema, underscoring the personalized nature of dietary responses.

The Symptom Spectrum of Wheat Intolerance

When addressing wheat intolerance, the symptoms can be as varied as the lengths of a string—unpredictable and wide-ranging. This variability emphasizes the importance of personal trial and error in identifying and managing triggers. It is a reminder that individuals must become advocates for their own health, adopting what benefits them and adjusting as needed.

The Role of Sunshine and Sea Water in Healing

Another case study highlights the therapeutic effects of natural elements. A child with eczema found relief by spending a summer by the sea, bathing in the ocean, and basking in the sun. While the sunshine provides significant benefits, it is cautioned to be enjoyed within reason, especially for those with light-sensitive skin or a a tendency to itch.

The Necessity of Ice for Inflammation

The chapter concludes by championing ice as a powerful anti-inflammatory tool, especially crucial for managing eczema. Scratching might offer temporary relief, yet it ultimately exacerbates inflammation. Ice, on the other hand, can provide lasting relief without the adverse effects of scratching.

Conclusion

Conquering psoriasis or eczema requires a multifaceted approach that includes environmental control, dietary management, and the strategic use of natural remedies. The importance of individualized care cannot be overstated, with each person needing to become their own investigator and healer, using discretion and patience on their path to recovery.

Chapter 7

THE PILLARS OF DIETARY TEMPERANCE FOR SKIN HEALTH

The Principle of Moderation in Managing Skin Conditions

Temperance is fundamental in addressing skin ailments such as eczema and psoriasis. It involves a dual approach: abstaining from harmful substances and consuming alternative beneficial items instead. This chapter delves into the practical application of moderation in diet and lifestyle for those afflicted with these conditions.

The Rigorous Elimination Phase

For individuals like Matthew, who has navigated the challenges of psoriasis, the initial phase of management is strict avoidance. Wheat, even in its ancient forms, dairy, oats, peanuts, and refined sugar are eliminated from the diet. Peanuts, in particular, are noted due to their propensity for mold contamination, highlighted in "The China Study," where aflatoxin presence was a significant concern.

The Gradual Reintroduction Strategy

Once control is gained, and skin health is restored, a careful reintroduction of certain foods, like ancient grains, can be considered. Matthew's own regime allows for an occasional slice of bread without adverse effects, but only spaced out over several days. This reintroduction phase embodies restraint in practice—moderation once healing has occurred.

The Role of Chemicals and Molds

The elimination of external triggers, particularly chemicals and molds, is equally crucial. Attention is turned to everyday items such as laundry detergents. The recommendation is to opt for biodegradable, environmentally-friendly detergents, or even simple sodium bicarbonate, to reduce potential skin irritants in clothing.

Clothing Considerations for Skin Health

The fabric that comes into contact with the skin is of paramount importance. Clothes should ideally be made from natural fibers like cotton, silk, wool, flax, hemp, and modern fibers like modal, viscose, and rayon, which are derived from wood pulp. Despite concerns about the chemical processes in manufacturing these materials, thorough washing and sun-drying can mitigate potential residue, harnessing the purifying power of the sun.

Thrift Shopping for Natural Fibers

The cost of natural fibers can be prohibitive; however, thrift stores present an economical and sustainable alternative. Often, higher quality natural cotton garments can be found second-hand, providing a skin-friendly wardrobe without the expense of new clothing.

Conclusion

This chapter emphasizes the importance of temperance in managing skin conditions. It outlines a comprehensive approach, from dietary restrictions to lifestyle adjustments, underscoring the necessity of natural, non-irritating materials in clothing. Through the practice of moderation, individuals like Matthew find a balance that allows them to manage their skin conditions effectively and sustainably.

Chapter 8

RESTORATIVE LIFESTYLE CHOICES FOR SKIN HEALTH

Embracing Restorative Sleep

Sleep is the fourth key pillar in managing skin conditions, acting as a time for the body to recharge and intensify its healing processes. For adults, 8 hours of sleep is ideal, while children benefit from 10. Creating a conducive environment for sleep is essential—low lighting, a substantial midday meal followed by a lighter evening meal, soft music, and a relaxing bedtime story can help ease children into an early bedtime. Adults, too, can retrain their brains to embrace a full night's rest, ultimately feeling the benefits of extended sleep.

The Role of Exercise

Exercise, the fifth element, is critical for overall health and particularly beneficial for those with psoriasis. Swimming in the ocean is recommended due to the cooling effects of the water, which can prevent overheating and irritation of the skin. For those without access to the ocean, exercises such as cycling or rebounding, followed by a cold shower, can provide the necessary physical activity without exacerbating skin conditions.

Revising Dietary Habits

When it comes to diet, the need for modification becomes apparent upon the elimination of irritants such as wheat and dairy. Alternative grains like millet, quinoa, and rice offer safe and satisfying options. These grains can be prepared in various ways to ensure digestibility and enjoyment. Sweetening agents like honey, maple syrup, and palm sugar, along with a range of nut butters, offer healthier alternatives to refined sugars and peanuts.

The Importance of Protein and Fats

Protein is a vital component of the diet, with legumes serving as a substantial source. Preparing these in bulk and freezing portions can provide convenient and tasty meals. When it comes to fats, they are essential for maintaining the cellular structure, with natural sources such as nuts and seeds being highly recommended.

Supper Considerations

For supper, light and savory meals are preferable. Sugary foods should be limited to avoid exacerbating skin irritation. Herbal teas or smoothies made with coconut water or almond milk can be enriched with chia and flaxseeds, which are high in omega-3 fatty acids and provide internal nourishment for the skin.

Hydration as a Keystone of Health

Finally, hydration cannot be overstated in its importance. Drinking adequate water is vital for the body's nighttime rejuvenation processes. Ensuring that the digestive system is at rest during sleep allows the body's energy to focus on healing and revitalization.

Conclusion

This chapter outlines a comprehensive approach to managing skin conditions through lifestyle adjustments. Prioritizing restorative sleep, engaging in appropriate exercise, revising diet to eliminate irritants and embrace healthy alternatives, and ensuring proper hydration all play crucial roles in supporting the body's natural healing mechanisms. By adopting these practices, individuals can create a conducive environment for skin health and overall well-being.

Chapter 9

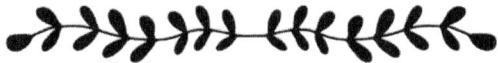

HYDRATION AND TRUST AS CORNERSTONES OF HEALING

The Vitality of Water for Skin Health

Hydration is pivotal in maintaining skin suppleness and health. The "rule of thumb" for water intake is approximately one quart per 50 pounds of body weight. This formula aids in determining the appropriate amount for both adults and children. To ensure adequate hydration throughout the day, one can follow a routine of drinking water at regular intervals, starting from the morning and before engaging in exercise, with a mindful reduction in the evening to prevent nocturnal disruptions.

The Significance of Salt

In addition to water, the inclusion of whole salts, like Celtic or Himalayan salt, is essential for maintaining the body's electrolyte balance. These should be consumed in small amounts throughout the day to complement the body's hydration needs.

Trust in Divine Power for Stress Management

The eighth law discussed is trust in divine power. Stress has been recognized as a significant exacerbator of skin conditions like eczema. Embracing a daily practice of trust and gratitude, as encouraged by scriptural references, can have a profound impact on stress levels and overall well-being. The philosophy here is to live in the present moment, appreciating today's gift and trusting in divine guidance for tomorrow.

Internal Medicine Through Nutrition

Addressing the body's internal environment is crucial for managing skin conditions. Foods high in fiber, protein, and healthy fats form the triad of internal medicine. Seeds like chia and flax, rich in omega-3 fatty acids, are particularly emphasized for their skin-nourishing properties. They can be integrated into meals in various forms, from sprinkled on breakfast cereals to incorporated into snackable date and nut balls.

Proper Fats for Skin Nourishment

Healthy fats, such as those found in nuts, seeds, olive oil, and coconut, are vital for skin health. They form the cellular membrane and provide essential nourishment from within. Regular incorporation of these fats into the diet, through both cooking and direct addition to meals, ensures that the skin receives the necessary nutrients to maintain its integrity and function.

Conclusion

This chapter highlights the importance of hydration and stress management as integral components of skin health. It also underscores the significance of nutrition as internal medicine, with a focus on foods that provide the necessary fiber, protein, and fats. By adopting these principles, individuals can support their body's natural healing processes and improve conditions like eczema and psoriasis from the inside out.

Chapter 10

LIVER HEALTH AND ELIMINATION PATHWAYS IN SKIN HEALING

The Liver's Role in Detoxification and Skin Health

The liver, described as the body's orchestrator, plays a critical role in detoxification, particularly when the body is exposed to mold and chemicals. Herbs such as dandelion and milk thistle are highlighted for their liver-supporting properties. These can be incorporated into the diet through salads or taken in supplement form to aid in the detoxifying process and, consequently, skin healing.

Dandelion and Milk Thistle for Liver Support

Dandelion, often found growing wild, can be finely sliced and added to salads, providing a bitter counterpoint to sweeter vegetables. Milk Thistle, or St. Mary's Thistle, is known for its potent liver-boosting effects. Gentian, a lesser-known root, is also mentioned for its bitter, liver-supportive properties. These herbs, due to their bitterness, are sometimes preferred in tablet or capsule form to enhance liver function, which in turn supports skin health.

Lifestyle Choices and Skin Conditions

The narrative reinforces the notion that genetics may predispose one to skin conditions, but lifestyle choices trigger their manifestation. Alternatives to favorite foods that may exacerbate skin conditions are suggested, emphasizing that avoidance is not necessarily permanent but a temporary measure until healing occurs. After recovery, moderation and careful reintroduction of certain foods can be explored.

Elimination Organs in Detoxification

The skin, kidneys, and colon are identified as vital organs of elimination. Ensuring these pathways are functioning optimally is crucial for skin health. The skin benefits from natural fibers and soothing applications like aloe vera or coconut oil. Ice is also advocated as an effective method to calm inflammation and itchiness. For the kidneys, ample water intake is encouraged, with the amount adjusted according to body weight.

Encouraging Colon Health

Colon health is essential for elimination and can be supported by dietary choices such as the inclusion of chia and flax seeds, which help to stimulate bowel movements. The use of a 'squatty potty' or similar device can aid in a more natural and effective evacuation process.

A Case Study in Healing Psoriasis

The chapter concludes with a story of a man from Saudi Arabia who overcame severe, cortisone-treated psoriasis by stopping the cortisone cream and adopting a holistic approach, including juice fasting, liver herbs, and omega-3 rich seeds. Despite initial disappointment with the slow progress, he experienced a dramatic improvement six weeks later, showcasing the body's ability to heal itself over time when provided with the right conditions. This case also highlights the necessity to address environmental factors such as mold exposure, demonstrating the multifaceted approach required for skin healing.

Conclusion

Through an integrative approach focusing on liver health, elimination pathways, and trust in the body's inherent healing capacity, individuals can experience significant improvements in skin conditions such as eczema and psoriasis. This chapter underscores the importance of patience, persistence, and the power of natural remedies and lifestyle adjustments in the journey towards skin health and overall well-being.

Chapter 11

FUNDAMENTALS OF BALANCED NUTRITION: HARNESSING CARBOHYDRATES, PROTEINS, AND FATS FOR OPTIMAL HEALTH

When it comes to a balanced diet, it is essential to include a variety of macronutrients: carbohydrates, proteins, and fats. Each plays a vital role in maintaining health.

Carbohydrates:

Opt for complex carbohydrates that are full of fiber and low in added sugars. Ideal sources include:

- Whole Grains: Brown rice, millet, quinoa, and buckwheat are preferred for their nutritional completeness, providing fiber, vitamins, and minerals.

- Vegetables: Emphasize a rainbow of vegetables, with a focus on leafy greens for their nutrient density.

- Fruits: Choose fruits that are lower in sugars and higher in fiber, such as berries and apples, to be enjoyed in moderation.

- Legumes: Beans and lentils not only provide carbohydrates but are also excellent sources of protein and fiber.

Proteins:

Proteins are the building blocks of the body and are necessary for repair and growth. Include a variety of protein sources:

- Plant-Based Proteins: Foods like legumes, nuts, and seeds, along with whole grains, can provide adequate protein and other vital nutrients.

- Animal Proteins: If included in the diet, opt for options that are organic, free-range, or grass-fed to minimize exposure to antibiotics and hormones.

- Dairy Alternatives: Plant-based milks such as almond, soy, or coconut milk can serve as alternatives to traditional dairy, offering different nutritional profiles and benefits.

Fats:

Healthy fats are essential for brain health, energy, and cell structure. Incorporate healthy fats through:

- Unsaturated Fats: Avocados, nuts, and seeds are excellent sources and provide essential fatty acids.

- Omega-3 Fatty Acids: To support heart health and reduce inflammation, include flaxseeds, chia seeds, and hemp seeds in your diet.

- Minimally Processed Oils: Use oils like extra virgin olive oil for cold dishes or dressings and coconut oil for cooking at higher temperatures.

- Avoid Trans Fats: Steer clear of trans fats and hydrogenated oils commonly found in processed foods, as they can be harmful to cardiovascular health.

A diet rich in a variety of unprocessed foods, colorful vegetables, fiber-rich fruits, whole grains, and healthy fats can support overall well-being while providing necessary energy and nutrients for daily activities.

RECIPES: PROMOTING HEALTHY SKIN

These recipes are inspired by the principles of hydration, the importance of whole foods, and the avoidance of potential allergens and irritants as discussed in Barbara O'Neill's teachings. They emphasize natural, unprocessed ingredients and aim to support overall health and well-being.

These lists are tailored for preparing a single serving of each recipe. When purchasing ingredients like olive oil, tamari, or spices that you'll use across several recipes, you can buy standard-size containers as they have a long shelf life and can be used for multiple cooking sessions.

1. LUXURY MILLET PORRIDGE

Ingredients:
1. 1/4 cup millet
2. Honey or maple syrup (to taste)
3. A small handful of fresh berries (like raspberries, blueberries, or strawberries)
4. 1 teaspoon ground flaxseed

Instructions:
1. Rinse 1 cup of millet thoroughly in cold water.
2. In a medium saucepan, combine the rinsed millet with 4 cups of water.
3. Bring to a boil, then reduce the heat to a simmer. Cover and cook for 15-20 minutes or until the millet is soft and the water is absorbed.
4. Remove from heat and let it sit, covered, for 5 minutes.
5. Stir in a teaspoon of honey or maple syrup for sweetness.
6. Serve in bowls topped with fresh berries (such as raspberries, blueberries, or strawberries) and a sprinkle of ground flaxseed for added omega-3s.

2. QUINOA & ROASTED VEGETABLE SALAD

Ingredients:

1. 1/4 cup quinoa
2. 1/2 small zucchini
3. 1/2 bell pepper (any color)
4. 1/4 onion
5. Olive oil (for roasting and dressing)
6. Salt and pepper (to taste)
7. Fresh lemon juice (from 1/2 lemon)
8. Fresh parsley (a small handful)
9. 1 tablespoon hemp seeds

Instructions:

1. Preheat your oven to 400°F (200°C).
2. Cook 1 cup of quinoa according to package instructions and set aside to cool.
3. Chop a variety of vegetables (zucchini, bell peppers, onions) into bite-sized pieces and spread them on a baking sheet.
4. Drizzle the vegetables with olive oil and season with salt and pepper. Roast in the oven for about 25-30 minutes or until they are caramelized and tender.
5. In a large bowl, mix the roasted vegetables with the cooked quinoa.
6. Drizzle with olive oil and a squeeze of fresh lemon juice. Toss to combine.
7. Garnish with chopped parsley and a sprinkling of hemp seeds before serving.

3. LENTIL SOUP WITH KALE

Ingredients:

1. 1/4 cup green lentils
2. 1/2 carrot
3. 1/4 onion
4. 1 clove garlic
5. 1 1/2 cups vegetable broth
6. A small handful of kale leaves
7. Olive oil (for sautéing)
8. Salt and pepper (to taste)
9. A pinch of dried thyme

Instructions:

1. In a large pot, sauté 1 diced onion, 2 minced garlic cloves, and 2 diced carrots in a splash of olive oil until softened.
2. Pour in 6 cups of vegetable broth and 1 cup of rinsed green lentils.
3. Bring to a boil, then reduce to a simmer.
4. Add a bunch of kale, stemmed and chopped.
5. Season the soup with salt, pepper, and a pinch of dried thyme. Simmer for about 30 minutes or until the lentils are cooked through.
6. Serve the soup warm, adjusting seasoning to taste.

4. BUCKWHEAT NOODLE STIR-FRY

Ingredients:
1. 1 serving buckwheat noodles
2. 1/2 cup broccoli florets
3. 1/2 cup snap peas
4. 1/2 carrot, sliced
5. Olive oil (for stir-frying)
6. 1/2 tablespoon tamari or soy sauce
7. 1/4 teaspoon grated ginger
8. 1 clove garlic, minced

Instructions:
1. Cook buckwheat noodles according to package instructions, then drain and set aside.
2. In a wok or large frying pan, stir-fry a mixture of vegetables (broccoli florets, snap peas, sliced carrots) in a bit of olive oil until just tender.
3. In a small bowl, whisk together 2 tablespoons of tamari, 1 teaspoon of grated ginger, and 1 minced garlic clove.
4. Add the cooked noodles to the vegetables in the pan, pour the sauce over the top, and toss everything to combine and heat through.
5. Serve the stir-fry warm.

5. CHICKPEA SALAD WRAP

Ingredients:

1. 1/2 cup cooked chickpeas (or half a can, drained and rinsed)
2. 1/4 celery stalk, diced
3. 1 tablespoon diced onion
4. Vegan mayo (enough to coat the mixture)
5. Salt and pepper (to taste)
6. 1 large lettuce leaf or 1 whole grain tortilla
7. 1/4 avocado, sliced

Instructions:

1. In a bowl, mash 1 can of drained and rinsed chickpeas with a fork.
2. Mix in 1 diced celery stalk, 1/4 diced onion, and enough vegan mayo to coat.
3. Season with salt and pepper to taste.
4. Lay out large lettuce leaves or whole grain tortillas.
5. Spoon the chickpea mixture onto the leaves or tortillas, add avocado slices, and roll up to serve.

6. EXOTIC RICE PUDDING

Ingredients:
1. 1/4 cup brown rice
2. 1/4 cup water
3. 1/4 cup coconut milk
4. A pinch of cinnamon
5. A drizzle of maple syrup
6. A few diced pieces of mango or pineapple

Instructions:
1. In a saucepan, combine 1 cup of brown rice with 1 cup of water and 1 cup of coconut milk.
2. Bring to a boil, then reduce heat to a low simmer. Cover and cook until the rice is tender and the liquid is mostly absorbed, about 45 minutes.
3. Stir in a pinch of cinnamon and a drizzle of maple syrup to sweeten.
4. Serve warm, topped with diced mango or pineapple.

7. VEGETARIAN CHILI

Ingredients:

1. 1/4 can black beans
2. 1/4 can kidney beans
3. 1/2 can diced tomatoes
4. 1/4 onion, diced
5. 1 clove garlic, minced
6. 1/4 bell pepper, diced
7. 1/4 teaspoon ground cumin
8. 1/4 teaspoon chili powder
9. 1/8 teaspoon paprika
10. Salt (to taste)
11. A small handful of cilantro, chopped
12. 1/4 avocado, diced

Instructions:

1. In a large pot, sauté 1 diced onion, 2 minced garlic cloves, and 1 diced bell pepper in olive oil until soft.
2. Add 1 can of drained black beans, 1 can of drained kidney beans, and 1 can of diced tomatoes with their juice.
3. Stir in 1 teaspoon of ground cumin, 1 teaspoon of chili powder, and 1/2 teaspoon of paprika.
4. Bring to a simmer and cook for at least 30 minutes, stirring occasionally.
5. Serve hot, garnished with diced avocado and chopped fresh cilantro.

8. BAKED SWEET POTATO WITH SPINACH AND MACADAMIA NUTS

Ingredients:
1. 1 small sweet potato
2. Olive oil (for drizzling)
3. Celtic salt (to taste)
4. 1/2 cup spinach
5. 1 tablespoon crushed macadamia nuts

Instructions:
1. Preheat the oven to 400°F (200°C).
2. Prick the sweet potatoes with a fork and place them on a baking sheet.
3. Bake for about 45 minutes to 1 hour, or until tender.
4. Slice the sweet potatoes open and drizzle with olive oil.
5. Season with Celtic salt and top with sautéed spinach and crushed macadamia nuts.

9. ALMOND BUTTER & BANANA SMOOTHIE

Ingredients:
1. 1 small banana
2. 3/4 cup almond milk
3. 1/2 tablespoon almond butter
4. A dash of cinnamon
5. 1/2 teaspoon ground flaxseed
6. 1/2 teaspoon chia seeds

Instructions:
1. In a blender, combine 2 ripe bananas, 1 cup of almond milk, and 1 tablespoon of almond butter.
2. Add a dash of cinnamon and blend until smooth.
3. Pour into glasses and stir in 1 teaspoon each of ground flaxseed and chia seeds for extra nutrients.

10. CANNELLINI BEAN & VEGETABLE STEW

Ingredients:

1. 1/2 can cannellini beans
2. 1/2 can diced tomatoes
3. 1 cup vegetable broth
4. 1/4 onion, diced
5. 1 clove garlic, minced
6. A small amount of zucchini, chopped
7. A small amount of carrot, chopped
8. A small handful of kale, chopped
9. Italian herbs (to taste)
10. Olive oil (for sautéing)

Instructions:

1. Sauté 1 diced onion and 2 minced garlic cloves in a large pot with a bit of olive oil until translucent.
2. Add 1 can of drained cannellini beans, 1 can of diced tomatoes, and enough vegetable broth to cover the ingredients.
3. Add a variety of chopped vegetables (zucchini, carrots) and a handful of chopped kale.
4. Season with Italian herbs and simmer until the vegetables are tender.
5. Serve hot, with a side of whole grain bread for dipping.

These recipes embrace whole foods and are tailored to support skin health as per Barbara O'Neill's teachings. Enjoy the natural flavors and health benefits with each homemade meal.

Barbara O'Neill emphasizes the use of natural and non-toxic ingredients in daily life, including cleaning products. Here's a simple recipe for a natural washing powder that follows her principles:

11. NATURAL WASHING POWDER RECIPE

Ingredients:

1. 1 bar of pure castile soap or any unscented, natural soap
2. 1 cup of washing soda (sodium carbonate)
3. 1 cup of borax (sodium borate) - Note: Some people may prefer to avoid borax as it can be irritating to sensitive skin. For a borax-free version, you can just omit this ingredient.
4. 1 cup of baking soda (sodium bicarbonate)

Instructions:

1. Grate the Soap: Use a cheese grater to finely grate the bar of natural soap.
2. Mix the Powders: In a large bowl, mix the grated soap, washing soda, borax (if using), and baking soda together until well combined.
3. Blend for Finer Texture (Optional): For a finer texture, pulse the mixture in a food processor or blender. This helps the powder dissolve better in the washing machine, especially in cold water.
4. Store Properly: Transfer the washing powder to an airtight container to keep it dry and clump-free. Label the container for easy identification.
5. Use the Right Amount: Use 1-2 tablespoons of the washing powder per load, depending on the size and soil level of the laundry.

Tips and Considerations:

- If you have hard water, you may want to add a little more washing soda to the mixture to boost its effectiveness.

- For fragrance, consider adding a few drops of your favorite essential oil to the mix. Lavender, lemon, or eucalyptus are popular choices and have natural antibacterial properties.

- Always test the powder on a small piece of fabric first to ensure it doesn't cause any reaction, especially if you have sensitive skin.

- If you're washing clothes that are particularly dirty, you can pre-treat stains with a paste made from the washing powder and a bit of water before adding them to the wash.

By using this natural washing powder, you're avoiding the harsh chemicals found in many commercial detergents that can be detrimental to both your health and the environment, staying true to Barbara O'Neill's teachings.

Barbara O'Neill advocates for natural, chemical-free alternatives for household products. Based on her teachings, here is a recipe for a natural fabric softener:

12. NATURAL FABRIC SOFTENER RECIPE

Ingredients:

1. 1 cup of distilled white vinegar
2. ¼ cup of baking soda
3. 10-15 drops of essential oil (e.g., lavender, eucalyptus, or lemon for their natural antibacterial properties and pleasant scent)
4. 2 cups of hot water

Instructions:

- Mix Vinegar and Water: In a large bowl, carefully mix the distilled white vinegar with the hot water.
- Add Baking Soda: Slowly add the baking soda to the vinegar and water mixture. Do this step slowly as the vinegar and baking soda will react and fizz.
- Add Essential Oils: Once the fizzing has settled down, add your choice of essential oils to the mixture for a natural fragrance.
- Stir Gently: Stir the mixture gently to ensure all the ingredients are well combined.
- Transfer to Container: Pour the mixture into a large container with a lid, such as a gallon-sized jug or a repurposed fabric softener bottle.
- Use in Laundry: Shake well before each use. Add ¼ to ½ cup of the natural fabric softener to the rinse cycle of your wash. For smaller loads, you can reduce the amount accordingly.

Notes:

- Vinegar is a natural softening agent that can help to remove detergent residues and mineral build-up from fabrics.
- Baking soda softens the water, which can help fabrics to feel softer.
- Essential oils not only add fragrance but can also have additional properties like reducing static cling.
- This natural fabric softener can be safely used with most fabrics, but it's always wise to do a spot test if you're concerned about any materials.
- Avoid using this fabric softener on garments that are flame-resistant, as vinegar can break down the added flame-resistant properties.

By using this natural fabric softener, you are likely to avoid the chemicals and synthetic fragrances found in many commercial softeners, which aligns with the natural living principles that Barbara O'Neill encourages.

13. NATURAL TOOTHPASTE RECIPE

Ingredients:

1. 2 tablespoons of coconut oil (acts as a base and has antibacterial properties)
2. 2 tablespoons of baking soda (a gentle abrasive that helps clean and whiten teeth)
3. 10-15 drops of peppermint essential oil (for fresh breath; anti-bacterial)
4. 1 teaspoon of xylitol powder (optional, for sweetness and to combat harmful bacteria)
5. 1 teaspoon of bentonite clay (optional, for added minerals and detoxifying properties)

Instructions:

1. Prepare the Base: In a small bowl, mix the coconut oil and baking soda to form a paste. If the coconut oil is solid, you may gently warm it to a soft consistency but not liquid.
2. Add Essential Oils: Add the peppermint essential oil to the mixture. This not only provides a fresh minty flavor but also contributes to oral hygiene due to its antibacterial properties.
3. Sweeten Optionally: If desired, mix in the xylitol powder. Xylitol is known to be a dental-friendly sweetener and can help to reduce cavities.
4. Enrich with Clay: For an optional boost, gently fold in the bentonite clay. This natural clay can help remineralize teeth and absorb toxins.
5. Combine Thoroughly: Stir all the ingredients until you achieve a uniform paste. Ensure there are no lumps and that the texture is consistent.

6. Store Correctly: Transfer the paste into a small jar with a lid. To use, simply scoop a small amount onto your toothbrush with a spoon or spatula.

Notes:

- Coconut oil can solidify at cooler temperatures, so if you live in a cold climate, you might want to keep your toothpaste in a warm spot of your bathroom, or you may need to soften it slightly before use.

- Baking soda has a salty taste that some may not prefer; starting with a smaller amount and adjusting to taste can help.

- Peppermint essential oil should be food-grade quality to ensure safety for oral use.

- Always check for allergies or sensitivities to any of the ingredients before using the toothpaste regularly.

This natural toothpaste recipe avoids fluoride and other common commercial toothpaste additives, which is in line with Barbara O'Neill's teachings on natural health practices. It provides a simple, cost-effective, and health-conscious alternative to store-bought toothpastes.

14. SOOTHING NATURAL BODY BUTTER FOR ECZEMA

Ingredients:

- ½ cup shea butter (excellent for hydration and contains natural vitamins and fatty acids)
- ¼ cup coconut oil (has anti-inflammatory and moisturizing properties)
- ¼ cup almond oil (rich in Vitamin E, which can support skin healing)
- 1 tablespoon beeswax (helps to protect and repair the skin)
- 10-15 drops of lavender essential oil (known for its skin-soothing and anti-inflammatory properties)
- 5-10 drops of chamomile essential oil (optional, can help calm irritated skin)

Instructions:

1. Melt the Base: In a double boiler, gently melt the shea butter, coconut oil, and beeswax together until fully liquid.
2. Add Oils: Remove the mixture from heat and let it cool slightly. Then, stir in the almond oil.
3. Essential Oils: Once the mixture is just warm to the touch, add the lavender and chamomile essential oils. These oils are chosen for their soothing and anti-inflammatory properties, which are beneficial for eczema.
4. Chill: Place the mixture in the refrigerator for about 10-15 minutes or until it starts to solidify but is still somewhat soft.

5. Whip It: Using a hand mixer or stand mixer, whip the semi-solid mixture until it becomes fluffy and butter-like in texture.
6. Store: Transfer the whipped body butter into a clean, airtight glass jar for storage.
7. Use: Apply a small amount of the body butter to the affected areas of the skin. Use sparingly, as a little goes a long way.

Notes:

- Shea butter is a natural fat that is exceptionally good for dry and eczema-prone skin due to its moisturizing and healing properties.

- Coconut oil is used in this recipe for its skin-soothing benefits but should be patch tested first, as some individuals with eczema may find it irritating.

- Almond oil is generally well-tolerated by sensitive skin, but if you have a nut allergy, you can substitute it with another skin-friendly oil like jojoba or sunflower oil.

- Always do a patch test before applying new products to eczema-prone skin to ensure there is no reaction.

- If your eczema is severe or you are unsure about trying a new product, it is best to consult with a healthcare professional.

This body butter aims to moisturize and soothe the skin naturally, which can be beneficial for those with eczema when used as part of a broader skin care regimen focused on reducing inflammation and avoiding irritants.

Certain herbal teas may help alleviate the symptoms of eczema by supporting the body's immune system, reducing inflammation, or aiding in detoxification. Here are some teas that are often recommended for eczema:

1. **Chamomile Tea**: Known for its anti-inflammatory properties, chamomile tea can soothe the skin and reduce irritation.

2. **Green Tea**: Rich in antioxidants, green tea can help reduce inflammation and may help prevent the damage that inflammation can cause to the skin.

3. **Oolong Tea**: Some studies suggest that oolong tea can improve skin conditions by reducing inflammation and allergic reactions due to its antioxidant properties.

4. **Peppermint Tea**: Peppermint has a cooling effect on the skin and can relieve itching and irritation associated with eczema.

5. **Nettle Tea**: Nettle is a natural antihistamine and anti-inflammatory, which can help reduce eczema symptoms related to allergies.

6. **Red Clover Tea**: Traditionally used for various skin conditions, red clover may help with inflammation and irritation.

7. **Licorice Root Tea**: Licorice root has a corticosteroid-like effect that can relieve itching and soothe the skin, but it should be used in moderation.

8. **Calendula Tea**: Calendula can help heal skin inflammation and promote tissue repair due to its anti-inflammatory and antimicrobial properties.

9. **Burdock Root Tea**: Burdock root is known for its blood-purifying properties, which can help clear up skin conditions.

10. **Dandelion Tea**: Dandelion is another herb that is believed to help detoxify the liver and blood, potentially benefiting skin health.

11. **Yellow Dock Tea**: Yellow dock has traditionally been used to treat skin conditions, possibly due to its antioxidant and anti-inflammatory properties.

12. **Rooibos Tea**: Rooibos, or African red bush tea, is high in antioxidants and may benefit the skin by fighting inflammation.

It's important to note that while these teas can support skin health, they are not a cure for eczema. They should be used as a complementary approach to a holistic treatment plan. Also, before trying new herbal remedies, it's crucial to consult with a healthcare professional, especially if you are pregnant, breastfeeding, or have existing health conditions. This will ensure that the teas do not interact with any medications you may be taking and are safe for your particular health situation.

A Holistic Approach to Eczema and Psoriasis

The book presents a holistic view of health, with a focus on natural healing and may reduce the symptoms of disease through lifestyle and dietary choices. Drawing on the expertise of Barbara O'Neill, a nutritionist and health educator, it emphasizes the importance of understanding the body's natural healing mechanisms and supporting them through nutrition, herbal remedies, and other natural methods.

Diet: Central to O'Neill's philosophy is the consumption of a plant-based diet rich in whole, unprocessed foods. She advocates for the inclusion of complex carbohydrates from sources like millet and quinoa, which provide sustained energy and essential nutrients. Legumes, nuts, and seeds are recommended for their protein content, crucial for the body's repair and maintenance. The book also highlights the role of healthy fats, including those from avocados and seeds, which are supportive for brain health and cellular integrity.

Herbal Remedies: The teachings also extend to the use of herbal teas and remedies that can support the body's functions. Herbs like chamomile and nettle are suggested for their calming properties, which may help alleviate symptoms of conditions like eczema.

Lifestyle: Adequate hydration, restful sleep, regular exercise, and stress management are pillars of the recommended lifestyle. O'Neill advises on the careful management of stress through practices like meditation and spending time in nature, which can have profound effects on overall well-being and skin health.

Natural Products: The book also delves into the preparation of natural home remedies and personal care products. Recipes for natural toothpaste, body butter, and fabric softeners are provided, emphasizing the avoidance of harsh chemicals and the use of natural ingredients like coconut oil, shea butter, and essential oils.

In summary, the book encapsulates Barbara O'Neill's approach to health, which is rooted in the belief that the body has an innate ability to heal itself when given the right conditions. By embracing a natural, nutrient-rich diet, utilizing herbal remedies, and adopting a healthful lifestyle, individuals can support their body's healing processes and achieve a greater sense of well-being.

A Holistic Approach to Eczema and Psoriasis

Hydration First: Start your day with a glass of water to hydrate your body and skin.

NOTES

Date: ___/___/___

_____
_____
_____
_____

MOOD

☐ Hopeful ☐ Angry ☐ Bored

☐ Inspired ☐ Anxious ☐ Tired

☐ Happy ☐ Sad ☐ _____

WATER INTAKE

U U U
U U U
U U U
U U U

				Weather
Sleep	☐ High	☐ Med	☐ Low	
Energy Level	☐ High	☐ Med	☐ Low	
Activity Level	☐ High	☐ Med	☐ Low	

FOOD INTAKE

Time	Food	Triggers/Reactions

D.M. Clarke

Nourish Wisely: Choose anti-inflammatory foods that nourish your skin from the inside out.

NOTES

Date: ___/___/___

_____
_____
_____
_____

M O O D

- ☐ Hopeful ☐ Angry ☐ Bored
- ☐ Inspired ☐ Anxious ☐ Tired
- ☐ Happy ☐ Sad ☐ _____

WATER INTAKE

U U U
U U U
U U U
U U U

Sleep	☐ High	☐ Med	☐ Low	**Weather**
Energy Level	☐ High	☐ Med	☐ Low	
Activity Level	☐ High	☐ Med	☐ Low	

FOOD INTAKE

Time	Food	Triggers/Reactions

A Holistic Approach to Eczema and Psoriasis

Nourish Wisely: Choose anti-inflammatory foods that nourish your skin from the inside out.

NOTES

Date: ___/___/___

_____
_____
_____
_____

MOOD

☐ Hopeful ☐ Angry ☐ Bored

☐ Inspired ☐ Anxious ☐ Tired

☐ Happy ☐ Sad ☐ _____

WATER INTAKE

U U U
U U U
U U U
U U U

Sleep	☐ High	☐ Med	☐ Low	Weather
Energy Level	☐ High	☐ Med	☐ Low	
Activity Level	☐ High	☐ Med	☐ Low	

FOOD INTAKE

Time	Food	Triggers/Reactions

Mindful Eating: Eat slowly, savor each bite, and be mindful of your body's signals.

NOTES

Date: ___/___/___

_____
_____
_____
_____

M O O D

- ☐ Hopeful   ☐ Angry   ☐ Bored
- ☐ Inspired ☐ Anxious ☐ Tired
- ☐ Happy   ☐ Sad   ☐ _____

WATER INTAKE

U U U
U U U
U U U
U U U

				Weather
Sleep	☐ High	☐ Med	☐ Low	
Energy Level	☐ High	☐ Med	☐ Low	
Activity Level	☐ High	☐ Med	☐ Low	

FOOD INTAKE

Time	Food	Triggers/Reactions

A Holistic Approach to Eczema and Psoriasis

Mindful Eating: Eat slowly, savor each bite, and be mindful of your body's signals.

NOTES

Date: ___/___/___

_____
_____
_____
_____

MOOD

- ☐ Hopeful   ☐ Angry   ☐ Bored
- ☐ Inspired ☐ Anxious ☐ Tired
- ☐ Happy   ☐ Sad   ☐ _____

WATER INTAKE

U U U
U U U
U U U
U U U

				Weather
Sleep	☐ High	☐ Med	☐ Low	
Energy Level	☐ High	☐ Med	☐ Low	
Activity Level	☐ High	☐ Med	☐ Low	

FOOD INTAKE

Time	Food	Triggers/Reactions

Balance Your Meals: Incorporate a variety of nutrients into each meal for balanced health.

NOTES

Date: ___/___/___

_____
_____
_____
_____

M O O D

- ☐ Hopeful   ☐ Angry   ☐ Bored
- ☐ Inspired   ☐ Anxious ☐ Tired
- ☐ Happy   ☐ Sad   ☐ _____

WATER INTAKE

U U U
U U U
U U U
U U U

				Weather
Sleep	☐ High	☐ Med	☐ Low	
Energy Level	☐ High	☐ Med	☐ Low	
Activity Level	☐ High	☐ Med	☐ Low	

FOOD INTAKE

Time	Food	Triggers/Reactions

A Holistic Approach to Eczema and Psoriasis

Balance Your Meals: Incorporate a variety of nutrients into each meal for balanced health.

NOTES

Date: ___/___/___

_____
_____
_____
_____

MOOD

☐ Hopeful ☐ Angry ☐ Bored

☐ Inspired ☐ Anxious ☐ Tired

☐ Happy ☐ Sad ☐ _____

WATER INTAKE

U U U
U U U
U U U
U U U

				Weather
Sleep	☐ High	☐ Med	☐ Low	
Energy Level	☐ High	☐ Med	☐ Low	
Activity Level	☐ High	☐ Med	☐ Low	

FOOD INTAKE

Time	Food	Triggers/Reactions

Herbal Support: Remember to include liver-supportive herbs in your diet today.

NOTES

Date: ___/___/___

_____
_____
_____
_____

MOOD

☐ Hopeful ☐ Angry ☐ Bored

☐ Inspired ☐ Anxious ☐ Tired

☐ Happy ☐ Sad ☐ _____

WATER INTAKE

U U U
U U U
U U U
U U U

Sleep	☐ High	☐ Med	☐ Low	**Weather**
Energy Level	☐ High	☐ Med	☐ Low	
Activity Level	☐ High	☐ Med	☐ Low	

FOOD INTAKE

Time	Food	Triggers/Reactions

A Holistic Approach to Eczema and Psoriasis

Herbal Support: Remember to include liver-supportive herbs in your diet today.

NOTES

Date: ___/___/___

_____
_____
_____
_____

MOOD

- ☐ Hopeful
- ☐ Angry
- ☐ Bored
- ☐ Inspired
- ☐ Anxious
- ☐ Tired
- ☐ Happy
- ☐ Sad
- ☐ _____

WATER INTAKE

U U U
U U U
U U U
U U U

				Weather
Sleep	☐ High	☐ Med	☐ Low	
Energy Level	☐ High	☐ Med	☐ Low	
Activity Level	☐ High	☐ Med	☐ Low	

FOOD INTAKE

Time	Food	Triggers/Reactions

Keep Moving: Engage in gentle, non-irritating exercise to promote circulation and skin health.

NOTES
Date: ___/___/___

_____
_____
_____
_____

MOOD

☐ Hopeful   ☐ Angry   ☐ Bored

☐ Inspired   ☐ Anxious   ☐ Tired

☐ Happy   ☐ Sad   ☐ _____

WATER INTAKE

U U U
U U U
U U U
U U U

Sleep	☐ High	☐ Med	☐ Low	Weather
Energy Level	☐ High	☐ Med	☐ Low	
Activity Level	☐ High	☐ Med	☐ Low	

FOOD INTAKE

Time	Food	Triggers/Reactions

A Holistic Approach to Eczema and Psoriasis

Keep Moving: Engage in gentle, non-irritating exercise to promote circulation and skin health.

NOTES

Date: ___/___/___

_____
_____
_____
_____

MOOD

☐ Hopeful ☐ Angry ☐ Bored

☐ Inspired ☐ Anxious ☐ Tired

☐ Happy ☐ Sad ☐ _____

WATER INTAKE

U U U
U U U
U U U
U U U

Sleep	☐ High	☐ Med	☐ Low	**Weather**
Energy Level	☐ High	☐ Med	☐ Low	
Activity Level	☐ High	☐ Med	☐ Low	

FOOD INTAKE

Time	Food	Triggers/Reactions

Sunshine Sparingly: Get a moderate amount of sunlight for natural vitamin D, but don't overdo it.

NOTES

Date: ___/___/___

_____
_____
_____
_____

MOOD

☐ Hopeful   ☐ Angry   ☐ Bored

☐ Inspired   ☐ Anxious ☐ Tired

☐ Happy   ☐ Sad   ☐ _____

WATER INTAKE

U U U
U U U
U U U
U U U

Sleep	☐ High	☐ Med	☐ Low	**Weather**
Energy Level	☐ High	☐ Med	☐ Low	
Activity Level	☐ High	☐ Med	☐ Low	

FOOD INTAKE

Time	Food	Triggers/Reactions

Sunshine Sparingly: Get a moderate amount of sunlight for natural vitamin D, but don't overdo it.

NOTES

Date: ___/___/___

_____
_____
_____
_____

MOOD

- ☐ Hopeful   ☐ Angry   ☐ Bored
- ☐ Inspired ☐ Anxious ☐ Tired
- ☐ Happy   ☐ Sad   ☐ _____

WATER INTAKE

U U U
U U U
U U U
U U U

				Weather
Sleep	☐ High	☐ Med	☐ Low	
Energy Level	☐ High	☐ Med	☐ Low	
Activity Level	☐ High	☐ Med	☐ Low	

FOOD INTAKE

Time	Food	Triggers/Reactions

Rest and Digest: Take time to relax after meals for optimal digestion and absorption.

NOTES

Date: ___/___/___

_____
_____
_____
_____

MOOD

☐ Hopeful ☐ Angry ☐ Bored

☐ Inspired ☐ Anxious ☐ Tired

☐ Happy ☐ Sad ☐ _____

WATER INTAKE

U U U
U U U
U U U
U U U

Sleep	☐ High	☐ Med	☐ Low	Weather
Energy Level	☐ High	☐ Med	☐ Low	
Activity Level	☐ High	☐ Med	☐ Low	

FOOD INTAKE

Time	Food	Triggers/Reactions

Rest and Digest: Take time to relax after meals for optimal digestion and absorption.

NOTES

Date: ___/___/___

_____
_____
_____
_____

MOOD

☐ Hopeful   ☐ Angry   ☐ Bored

☐ Inspired   ☐ Anxious   ☐ Tired

☐ Happy   ☐ Sad   ☐ _____

WATER INTAKE

⋃ ⋃ ⋃
⋃ ⋃ ⋃
⋃ ⋃ ⋃
⋃ ⋃ ⋃

Sleep	☐ High	☐ Med	☐ Low	Weather
Energy Level	☐ High	☐ Med	☐ Low	
Activity Level	☐ High	☐ Med	☐ Low	

FOOD INTAKE

Time	Food	Triggers/Reactions

Skin-Friendly Fabrics: Wear natural fibers to let your skin breathe and prevent irritation.

NOTES
Date: ___/___/___

_____
_____
_____
_____

MOOD

- ☐ Hopeful   ☐ Angry   ☐ Bored
- ☐ Inspired   ☐ Anxious ☐ Tired
- ☐ Happy   ☐ Sad   ☐ _____

WATER INTAKE

U U U
U U U
U U U
U U U

Sleep	☐ High	☐ Med	☐ Low	**Weather**
Energy Level	☐ High	☐ Med	☐ Low	
Activity Level	☐ High	☐ Med	☐ Low	

FOOD INTAKE

Time	Food	Triggers/Reactions

A Holistic Approach to Eczema and Psoriasis

Skin-Friendly Fabrics: Wear natural fibers to let your skin breathe and prevent irritation.

NOTES

Date: ___/___/___

_____
_____
_____
_____

MOOD

- ☐ Hopeful   ☐ Angry   ☐ Bored
- ☐ Inspired   ☐ Anxious   ☐ Tired
- ☐ Happy   ☐ Sad   ☐ _____

WATER INTAKE

U U U
U U U
U U U
U U U

				Weather
Sleep	☐ High	☐ Med	☐ Low	
Energy Level	☐ High	☐ Med	☐ Low	
Activity Level	☐ High	☐ Med	☐ Low	

FOOD INTAKE

Time	Food	Triggers/Reactions

D.M. Clarke

Stay Positive: Keep a positive mindset; your attitude can influence your skin's health.

NOTES

Date: ___/___/___

_____
_____
_____
_____

MOOD

☐ Hopeful   ☐ Angry   ☐ Bored

☐ Inspired   ☐ Anxious   ☐ Tired

☐ Happy   ☐ Sad   ☐ _____

WATER INTAKE

U U U
U U U
U U U
U U U

				Weather
Sleep	☐ High	☐ Med	☐ Low	
Energy Level	☐ High	☐ Med	☐ Low	
Activity Level	☐ High	☐ Med	☐ Low	

FOOD INTAKE

Time	Food	Triggers/Reactions

A Holistic Approach to Eczema and Psoriasis

Stay Positive: Keep a positive mindset; your attitude can influence your skin's health.

NOTES

Date: ___/___/___

_____
_____
_____
_____

MOOD

☐ Hopeful ☐ Angry ☐ Bored

☐ Inspired ☐ Anxious ☐ Tired

☐ Happy ☐ Sad ☐ _____

WATER INTAKE

U U U
U U U
U U U
U U U

Sleep	☐ High	☐ Med	☐ Low	Weather
Energy Level	☐ High	☐ Med	☐ Low	
Activity Level	☐ High	☐ Med	☐ Low	

FOOD INTAKE

Time	Food	Triggers/Reactions

D.M. Clarke

Sleep Soundly: Ensure you get enough rest; sleep is when your skin repairs itself.

NOTES

Date: ___/___/___

_____
_____
_____
_____

MOOD

☐ Hopeful   ☐ Angry   ☐ Bored

☐ Inspired   ☐ Anxious   ☐ Tired

☐ Happy   ☐ Sad   ☐ _____

WATER INTAKE

U U U
U U U
U U U
U U U

				Weather
Sleep	☐ High	☐ Med	☐ Low	
Energy Level	☐ High	☐ Med	☐ Low	
Activity Level	☐ High	☐ Med	☐ Low	

FOOD INTAKE

Time	Food	Triggers/Reactions

Sleep Soundly: Ensure you get enough rest; sleep is when your skin repairs itself.

NOTES   Date: ___/___/___

_____
_____
_____
_____

M O O D

☐ Hopeful   ☐ Angry   ☐ Bored

☐ Inspired   ☐ Anxious   ☐ Tired

☐ Happy   ☐ Sad   ☐ _____

WATER INTAKE

U U U
U U U
U U U
U U U

Sleep	☐ High	☐ Med	☐ Low	**Weather**
Energy Level	☐ High	☐ Med	☐ Low	
Activity Level	☐ High	☐ Med	☐ Low	

FOOD INTAKE

Time	Food	Triggers/Reactions

D.M. Clarke

Stress Less: Find ways to manage stress, whether through meditation, reading, or a hobby.

NOTES

Date: ___/___/___

_____
_____
_____
_____

M O O D

- ☐ Hopeful   ☐ Angry   ☐ Bored
- ☐ Inspired ☐ Anxious ☐ Tired
- ☐ Happy   ☐ Sad   ☐ _____

WATER INTAKE

U U U
U U U
U U U
U U U

				Weather
Sleep	☐ High	☐ Med	☐ Low	
Energy Level	☐ High	☐ Med	☐ Low	
Activity Level	☐ High	☐ Med	☐ Low	

FOOD INTAKE

Time	Food	Triggers/Reactions

A Holistic Approach to Eczema and Psoriasis

Stress Less: Find ways to manage stress, whether through meditation, reading, or a hobby.

NOTES

Date: ___/___/___

_____
_____
_____
_____

MOOD

- ☐ Hopeful   ☐ Angry   ☐ Bored
- ☐ Inspired ☐ Anxious ☐ Tired
- ☐ Happy   ☐ Sad   ☐ _____

WATER INTAKE

U U U
U U U
U U U
U U U

				Weather
Sleep	☐ High	☐ Med	☐ Low	
Energy Level	☐ High	☐ Med	☐ Low	
Activity Level	☐ High	☐ Med	☐ Low	

FOOD INTAKE

Time	Food	Triggers/Reactions

D.M. Clarke

Stay Cool: Avoid hot showers and baths which can irritate your skin. Opt for lukewarm water.

NOTES   Date: ___/___/___

_____
_____
_____
_____

MOOD

☐ Hopeful   ☐ Angry   ☐ Bored

☐ Inspired   ☐ Anxious   ☐ Tired

☐ Happy   ☐ Sad   ☐ _____

WATER INTAKE

U U U
U U U
U U U
U U U

Sleep	☐ High	☐ Med	☐ Low	Weather
Energy Level	☐ High	☐ Med	☐ Low	
Activity Level	☐ High	☐ Med	☐ Low	

FOOD INTAKE

Time	Food	Triggers/Reactions

A Holistic Approach to Eczema and Psoriasis

Stay Cool: Avoid hot showers and baths which can irritate your skin. Opt for lukewarm water.

NOTES

Date: ___/___/___

_____
_____
_____
_____

MOOD

☐ Hopeful ☐ Angry ☐ Bored

☐ Inspired ☐ Anxious ☐ Tired

☐ Happy ☐ Sad ☐ _____

WATER INTAKE

U U U
U U U
U U U
U U U

				Weather
Sleep	☐ High	☐ Med	☐ Low	
Energy Level	☐ High	☐ Med	☐ Low	
Activity Level	☐ High	☐ Med	☐ Low	

FOOD INTAKE

Time	Food	Triggers/Reactions

Hydration Throughout: Keep sipping water all day to maintain skin hydration.

NOTES

Date: ___/___/___

_____
_____
_____
_____

MOOD

☐ Hopeful ☐ Angry ☐ Bored

☐ Inspired ☐ Anxious ☐ Tired

☐ Happy ☐ Sad ☐ _____

WATER INTAKE

U U U
U U U
U U U
U U U

Sleep	☐ High	☐ Med	☐ Low	Weather
Energy Level	☐ High	☐ Med	☐ Low	
Activity Level	☐ High	☐ Med	☐ Low	

FOOD INTAKE

Time	Food	Triggers/Reactions

A Holistic Approach to Eczema and Psoriasis

Hydration Throughout: Keep sipping water all day to maintain skin hydration.

NOTES

Date: ___/___/___

_____
_____
_____
_____

MOOD

☐ Hopeful ☐ Angry ☐ Bored

☐ Inspired ☐ Anxious ☐ Tired

☐ Happy ☐ Sad ☐ _____

WATER INTAKE

U U U
U U U
U U U
U U U

				Weather
Sleep	☐ High	☐ Med	☐ Low	
Energy Level	☐ High	☐ Med	☐ Low	
Activity Level	☐ High	☐ Med	☐ Low	

FOOD INTAKE

Time	Food	Triggers/Reactions

D.M. Clarke

Detox Daily: Support your body's natural detoxification processes w with the right foods and habits.

NOTES

Date: ___/___/___

_____
_____
_____
_____

MOOD

☐ Hopeful   ☐ Angry   ☐ Bored

☐ Inspired   ☐ Anxious ☐ Tired

☐ Happy   ☐ Sad   ☐ _____

WATER INTAKE

U U U
U U U
U U U
U U U

				Weather
Sleep	☐ High	☐ Med	☐ Low	
Energy Level	☐ High	☐ Med	☐ Low	
Activity Level	☐ High	☐ Med	☐ Low	

FOOD INTAKE

Time	Food	Triggers/Reactions

A Holistic Approach to Eczema and Psoriasis

Detox Daily: Support your body's natural detoxification processes w with the right foods and habits.

NOTES   Date: ___/___/___

_____
_____
_____
_____

MOOD

- ☐ Hopeful   ☐ Angry   ☐ Bored
- ☐ Inspired   ☐ Anxious   ☐ Tired
- ☐ Happy   ☐ Sad   ☐ _____

WATER INTAKE

U U U
U U U
U U U
U U U

Sleep	☐ High	☐ Med	☐ Low	**Weather**
Energy Level	☐ High	☐ Med	☐ Low	
Activity Level	☐ High	☐ Med	☐ Low	

FOOD INTAKE

Time	Food	Triggers/Reactions

Go Green: Eat plenty of leafy greens for their skin-supporting antioxidants.

NOTES   Date: ___/___/___

_____
_____
_____
_____

MOOD

☐ Hopeful   ☐ Angry   ☐ Bored

☐ Inspired   ☐ Anxious   ☐ Tired

☐ Happy   ☐ Sad   ☐ _____

WATER INTAKE

U U U
U U U
U U U
U U U

				Weather
Sleep	☐ High	☐ Med	☐ Low	
Energy Level	☐ High	☐ Med	☐ Low	
Activity Level	☐ High	☐ Med	☐ Low	

FOOD INTAKE

Time	Food	Triggers/Reactions

A Holistic Approach to Eczema and Psoriasis

Go Green: Eat plenty of leafy greens for their skin-supporting antioxidants.

NOTES

Date: ___/___/___

MOOD

☐ Hopeful ☐ Angry ☐ Bored

☐ Inspired ☐ Anxious ☐ Tired

☐ Happy ☐ Sad ☐ _____

WATER INTAKE

U U U
U U U
U U U
U U U

				Weather
Sleep	☐ High	☐ Med	☐ Low	
Energy Level	☐ High	☐ Med	☐ Low	
Activity Level	☐ High	☐ Med	☐ Low	

FOOD INTAKE

Time	Food	Triggers/Reactions

Evening Wind-Down: Dim the lights and reduce screen time to prepare your body for rest.

NOTES

Date: ___/___/___

_____
_____
_____
_____

M O O D

☐ Hopeful   ☐ Angry   ☐ Bored

☐ Inspired   ☐ Anxious   ☐ Tired

☐ Happy   ☐ Sad   ☐ _____

WATER INTAKE

U U U
U U U
U U U
U U U

Sleep	☐ High	☐ Med	☐ Low
Energy Level	☐ High	☐ Med	☐ Low
Activity Level	☐ High	☐ Med	☐ Low

Weather

FOOD INTAKE

Time	Food	Triggers/Reactions

A Holistic Approach to Eczema and Psoriasis

Evening Wind-Down: Dim the lights and reduce screen time to prepare your body for rest.

NOTES

Date: ___/___/___

_____
_____
_____
_____

MOOD

- ☐ Hopeful   ☐ Angry   ☐ Bored
- ☐ Inspired ☐ Anxious ☐ Tired
- ☐ Happy   ☐ Sad   ☐ _____

WATER INTAKE

☐ ☐ ☐
☐ ☐ ☐
☐ ☐ ☐
☐ ☐ ☐

				Weather
Sleep	☐ High	☐ Med	☐ Low	
Energy Level	☐ High	☐ Med	☐ Low	
Activity Level	☐ High	☐ Med	☐ Low	

FOOD INTAKE

Time	Food	Triggers/Reactions

D.M. Clarke

Reflect Gratefully: End your day by noting something you're grateful for.

NOTES

Date: ___/___/___

_____
_____
_____
_____

MOOD

☐ Hopeful　　☐ Angry　　☐ Bored

☐ Inspired　　☐ Anxious　　☐ Tired

☐ Happy　　☐ Sad　　☐ _____

WATER INTAKE

U　U　U
U　U　U
U　U　U
U　U　U

Sleep	☐ High	☐ Med	☐ Low	**Weather**
Energy Level	☐ High	☐ Med	☐ Low	
Activity Level	☐ High	☐ Med	☐ Low	

FOOD INTAKE

Time	Food	Triggers/Reactions

A Holistic Approach to Eczema and Psoriasis

Reflect Gratefully: End your day by noting something you're grateful for.

NOTES Date: ___/___/___

_____
_____
_____
_____

M O O D

- ☐ Hopeful   ☐ Angry   ☐ Bored
- ☐ Inspired   ☐ Anxious ☐ Tired
- ☐ Happy   ☐ Sad   ☐ _____

WATER INTAKE

U U U
U U U
U U U
U U U

				Weather
Sleep	☐ High	☐ Med	☐ Low	
Energy Level	☐ High	☐ Med	☐ Low	
Activity Level	☐ High	☐ Med	☐ Low	

FOOD INTAKE

Time	Food	Triggers/Reactions

Track Progress: Jot down any changes in your skin's condition to track what works for you.

NOTES

Date: ___/___/___

_____
_____
_____
_____

MOOD

☐ Hopeful　　☐ Angry　　☐ Bored

☐ Inspired　　☐ Anxious　　☐ Tired

☐ Happy　　☐ Sad　　☐ _____

WATER INTAKE

U　U　U
U　U　U
U　U　U
U　U　U

Sleep	☐ High	☐ Med	☐ Low
Energy Level	☐ High	☐ Med	☐ Low
Activity Level	☐ High	☐ Med	☐ Low

Weather

FOOD INTAKE

Time	Food	Triggers/Reactions

A Holistic Approach to Eczema and Psoriasis

Track Progress: Jot down any changes in your skin's condition to track what works for you.

NOTES Date: ___/___/___

_____

_____

_____

_____

MOOD

☐ Hopeful ☐ Angry ☐ Bored

☐ Inspired ☐ Anxious ☐ Tired

☐ Happy ☐ Sad ☐ _____

WATER INTAKE

U U U
U U U
U U U
U U U

Sleep	☐ High	☐ Med	☐ Low	**Weather**
Energy Level	☐ High	☐ Med	☐ Low	
Activity Level	☐ High	☐ Med	☐ Low	

FOOD INTAKE

Time	Food	Triggers/Reactions

Soothe with Ice: If itchiness arises, remember that ice can be a soothing remedy.

NOTES

Date: ___/___/___

_____
_____
_____
_____

MOOD

☐ Hopeful   ☐ Angry   ☐ Bored

☐ Inspired ☐ Anxious ☐ Tired

☐ Happy   ☐ Sad   ☐ _____

WATER INTAKE

U U U
U U U
U U U
U U U

Sleep	☐ High	☐ Med	☐ Low	**Weather**
Energy Level	☐ High	☐ Med	☐ Low	
Activity Level	☐ High	☐ Med	☐ Low	

FOOD INTAKE

Time	Food	Triggers/Reactions

A Holistic Approach to Eczema and Psoriasis

Soothe with Ice: If itchiness arises, remember that ice can be a soothing remedy.

NOTES   Date: ___/___/___

_____
_____
_____
_____

MOOD

- ☐ Hopeful   ☐ Angry   ☐ Bored
- ☐ Inspired   ☐ Anxious   ☐ Tired
- ☐ Happy   ☐ Sad   ☐ _____

WATER INTAKE

U U U
U U U
U U U
U U U

				Weather
Sleep	☐ High	☐ Med	☐ Low	
Energy Level	☐ High	☐ Med	☐ Low	
Activity Level	☐ High	☐ Med	☐ Low	

FOOD INTAKE

Time	Food	Triggers/Reactions

Less Is More: Use minimal, natural skincare products to avoid chemical irritants.

NOTES

Date: ___/___/___

_____
_____
_____
_____

MOOD

☐ Hopeful ☐ Angry ☐ Bored

☐ Inspired ☐ Anxious ☐ Tired

☐ Happy ☐ Sad ☐ _____

WATER INTAKE

U U U
U U U
U U U
U U U

Sleep	☐ High	☐ Med	☐ Low	**Weather**
Energy Level	☐ High	☐ Med	☐ Low	
Activity Level	☐ High	☐ Med	☐ Low	

FOOD INTAKE

Time	Food	Triggers/Reactions

A Holistic Approach to Eczema and Psoriasis

Less Is More: Use minimal, natural skincare products to avoid chemical irritants.

NOTES

Date: ___/___/___

_____
_____
_____
_____

MOOD

- ☐ Hopeful   ☐ Angry   ☐ Bored
- ☐ Inspired   ☐ Anxious   ☐ Tired
- ☐ Happy   ☐ Sad   ☐ _____

WATER INTAKE

U U U
U U U
U U U
U U U

				Weather
Sleep	☐ High	☐ Med	☐ Low	
Energy Level	☐ High	☐ Med	☐ Low	
Activity Level	☐ High	☐ Med	☐ Low	

FOOD INTAKE

Time	Food	Triggers/Reactions

Embrace Whole Foods: Focus on whole, unprocessed foods that are k kind to your skin.

NOTES

Date: ___/___/___

_____
_____
_____
_____

MOOD

☐ Hopeful ☐ Angry ☐ Bored

☐ Inspired ☐ Anxious ☐ Tired

☐ Happy ☐ Sad ☐ _____

WATER INTAKE

U U U
U U U
U U U
U U U

Sleep	☐ High	☐ Med	☐ Low	Weather
Energy Level	☐ High	☐ Med	☐ Low	
Activity Level	☐ High	☐ Med	☐ Low	

FOOD INTAKE

Time	Food	Triggers/Reactions

A Holistic Approach to Eczema and Psoriasis

Embrace Whole Foods: Focus on whole, unprocessed foods that are k kind to your skin.

NOTES

Date: ___/___/___

_____
_____
_____
_____

MOOD

- ☐ Hopeful   ☐ Angry   ☐ Bored
- ☐ Inspired   ☐ Anxious ☐ Tired
- ☐ Happy   ☐ Sad   ☐ _____

WATER INTAKE

U U U
U U U
U U U
U U U

				Weather
Sleep	☐ High	☐ Med	☐ Low	
Energy Level	☐ High	☐ Med	☐ Low	
Activity Level	☐ High	☐ Med	☐ Low	

FOOD INTAKE

Time	Food	Triggers/Reactions

D.M. Clarke

Be Patient: Healing takes time; be patient with your body and the process.

NOTES

Date: ___/___/___

_____
_____
_____
_____

MOOD

- ☐ Hopeful ☐ Angry ☐ Bored
- ☐ Inspired ☐ Anxious ☐ Tired
- ☐ Happy ☐ Sad ☐ _____

WATER INTAKE

U U U
U U U
U U U
U U U

				Weather
Sleep	☐ High	☐ Med	☐ Low	
Energy Level	☐ High	☐ Med	☐ Low	
Activity Level	☐ High	☐ Med	☐ Low	

FOOD INTAKE

Time	Food	Triggers/Reactions

A Holistic Approach to Eczema and Psoriasis

Be Patient: Healing takes time; be patient with your body and the process.

NOTES　　　　　　　　　　　　Date: ___/ ___/ ___

_____

_____

_____

_____

MOOD

☐ Hopeful　　☐ Angry　　☐ Bored

☐ Inspired　　☐ Anxious　　☐ Tired

☐ Happy　　☐ Sad　　☐ _____

WATER INTAKE

U　U　U
U　U　U
U　U　U
U　U　U

				Weather
Sleep	☐ High	☐ Med	☐ Low	
Energy Level	☐ High	☐ Med	☐ Low	
Activity Level	☐ High	☐ Med	☐ Low	

FOOD INTAKE

Time	Food	Triggers/Reactions

Limit Triggers: Avoid known irritants like dairy, refined sugar, and gluten.

NOTES

Date: ___/___/___

_____
_____
_____
_____

M O O D

☐ Hopeful   ☐ Angry   ☐ Bored

☐ Inspired ☐ Anxious ☐ Tired

☐ Happy   ☐ Sad   ☐ _____

WATER INTAKE

U U U
U U U
U U U
U U U

Sleep	☐ High	☐ Med	☐ Low
Energy Level	☐ High	☐ Med	☐ Low
Activity Level	☐ High	☐ Med	☐ Low

Weather

FOOD INTAKE

Time	Food	Triggers/Reactions

A Holistic Approach to Eczema and Psoriasis

Limit Triggers: Avoid known irritants like dairy, refined sugar, and gluten.

NOTES

Date: ___/___/___

_____
_____
_____
_____

MOOD

- ☐ Hopeful   ☐ Angry   ☐ Bored
- ☐ Inspired   ☐ Anxious   ☐ Tired
- ☐ Happy   ☐ Sad   ☐ _____

WATER INTAKE

U U U
U U U
U U U
U U U

				Weather
Sleep	☐ High	☐ Med	☐ Low	
Energy Level	☐ High	☐ Med	☐ Low	
Activity Level	☐ High	☐ Med	☐ Low	

FOOD INTAKE

Time	Food	Triggers/Reactions

Natural Clean: Use homemade natural cleaning products to reduce chemical exposure.

NOTES

Date: ___/___/___

_____
_____
_____
_____

MOOD

☐ Hopeful ☐ Angry ☐ Bored

☐ Inspired ☐ Anxious ☐ Tired

☐ Happy ☐ Sad ☐ _____

WATER INTAKE

U U U
U U U
U U U
U U U

Sleep	☐ High	☐ Med	☐ Low	Weather
Energy Level	☐ High	☐ Med	☐ Low	
Activity Level	☐ High	☐ Med	☐ Low	

FOOD INTAKE

Time	Food	Triggers/Reactions

A Holistic Approach to Eczema and Psoriasis

Natural Clean: Use homemade natural cleaning products to reduce chemical exposure.

NOTES

Date: ___/___/___

_____
_____
_____
_____

M O O D

- ☐ Hopeful ☐ Angry ☐ Bored
- ☐ Inspired ☐ Anxious ☐ Tired
- ☐ Happy ☐ Sad ☐ _____

WATER INTAKE

U U U
U U U
U U U
U U U

				Weather
Sleep	☐ High	☐ Med	☐ Low	
Energy Level	☐ High	☐ Med	☐ Low	
Activity Level	☐ High	☐ Med	☐ Low	

FOOD INTAKE

Time	Food	Triggers/Reactions

Calm with Tea: Drink herbal teas that promote relaxation and skin health.

NOTES

Date: ___/___/___

_____
_____
_____
_____

M O O D

☐ Hopeful   ☐ Angry   ☐ Bored

☐ Inspired   ☐ Anxious   ☐ Tired

☐ Happy   ☐ Sad   ☐ _____

WATER INTAKE

U U U
U U U
U U U
U U U

				Weather
Sleep	☐ High	☐ Med	☐ Low	
Energy Level	☐ High	☐ Med	☐ Low	
Activity Level	☐ High	☐ Med	☐ Low	

FOOD INTAKE

Time	Food	Triggers/Reactions

A Holistic Approach to Eczema and Psoriasis

Calm with Tea: Drink herbal teas that promote relaxation and skin health.

NOTES

Date: ___/___/___

_____

_____

_____

_____

MOOD

- ☐ Hopeful   ☐ Angry   ☐ Bored
- ☐ Inspired ☐ Anxious ☐ Tired
- ☐ Happy   ☐ Sad   ☐ _____

WATER INTAKE

U U U
U U U
U U U
U U U

				Weather
Sleep	☐ High	☐ Med	☐ Low	
Energy Level	☐ High	☐ Med	☐ Low	
Activity Level	☐ High	☐ Med	☐ Low	

FOOD INTAKE

Time	Food	Triggers/Reactions

Fresh Air Fix: Make time to get outside for fresh air and a change of environment.

NOTES
Date: ___/___/___

_____
_____
_____
_____

MOOD

☐ Hopeful ☐ Angry   ☐ Bored

☐ Inspired ☐ Anxious ☐ Tired

☐ Happy   ☐ Sad   ☐ _____

WATER INTAKE

U U U
U U U
U U U
U U U

				Weather
Sleep	☐ High	☐ Med	☐ Low	
Energy Level	☐ High	☐ Med	☐ Low	
Activity Level	☐ High	☐ Med	☐ Low	

FOOD INTAKE

Time	Food	Triggers/Reactions

Fresh Air Fix: Make time to get outside for fresh air and a change of environment.

NOTES

Date: ___/___/___

_____
_____
_____
_____

MOOD

☐ Hopeful ☐ Angry ☐ Bored

☐ Inspired ☐ Anxious ☐ Tired

☐ Happy ☐ Sad ☐ _____

WATER INTAKE

U U U
U U U
U U U
U U U

Sleep	☐ High	☐ Med	☐ Low	Weather
Energy Level	☐ High	☐ Med	☐ Low	
Activity Level	☐ High	☐ Med	☐ Low	

FOOD INTAKE

Time	Food	Triggers/Reactions

Optimize Elimination: Support your body's elimination pathways through diet and hydration.

NOTES

Date: ___/___/___

_____
_____
_____
_____

M O O D

☐ Hopeful ☐ Angry ☐ Bored

☐ Inspired ☐ Anxious ☐ Tired

☐ Happy ☐ Sad ☐ _____

WATER INTAKE

U U U
U U U
U U U
U U U

				Weather
Sleep	☐ High	☐ Med	☐ Low	
Energy Level	☐ High	☐ Med	☐ Low	
Activity Level	☐ High	☐ Med	☐ Low	

FOOD INTAKE

Time	Food	Triggers/Reactions

A Holistic Approach to Eczema and Psoriasis

Optimize Elimination: Support your body's elimination pathways through diet and hydration.

NOTES

Date: ___/___/___

_____
_____
_____
_____

MOOD

- ☐ Hopeful   ☐ Angry   ☐ Bored
- ☐ Inspired   ☐ Anxious ☐ Tired
- ☐ Happy   ☐ Sad   ☐ _____

WATER INTAKE

U U U
U U U
U U U
U U U

				Weather
Sleep	☐ High	☐ Med	☐ Low	
Energy Level	☐ High	☐ Med	☐ Low	
Activity Level	☐ High	☐ Med	☐ Low	

FOOD INTAKE

Time	Food	Triggers/Reactions

Cultivate Community: Connect with others for support, sharing experiences and tips.

NOTES

Date: ___/___/___

_____
_____
_____
_____

MOOD

- ☐ Hopeful   ☐ Angry   ☐ Bored
- ☐ Inspired ☐ Anxious ☐ Tired
- ☐ Happy   ☐ Sad   ☐ _____

WATER INTAKE

U U U
U U U
U U U
U U U

Sleep	☐ High	☐ Med	☐ Low	Weather
Energy Level	☐ High	☐ Med	☐ Low	
Activity Level	☐ High	☐ Med	☐ Low	

FOOD INTAKE

Time	Food	Triggers/Reactions

A Holistic Approach to Eczema and Psoriasis

Cultivate Community: Connect with others for support, sharing experiences and tips.

NOTES Date: ___/___/___

_____
_____
_____
_____

M O O D

- ☐ Hopeful   ☐ Angry   ☐ Bored
- ☐ Inspired   ☐ Anxious   ☐ Tired
- ☐ Happy   ☐ Sad   ☐ _____

WATER INTAKE

U U U
U U U
U U U
U U U

				Weather
Sleep	☐ High	☐ Med	☐ Low	
Energy Level	☐ High	☐ Med	☐ Low	
Activity Level	☐ High	☐ Med	☐ Low	

FOOD INTAKE

Time	Food	Triggers/Reactions

Self-Care Rituals: Make time for self-care rituals that promote relaxation and well-being.

NOTES

Date: ___/___/___

_____
_____
_____
_____

MOOD

- ☐ Hopeful ☐ Angry ☐ Bored
- ☐ Inspired ☐ Anxious ☐ Tired
- ☐ Happy ☐ Sad ☐ _____

WATER INTAKE

U U U
U U U
U U U
U U U

				Weather
Sleep	☐ High	☐ Med	☐ Low	
Energy Level	☐ High	☐ Med	☐ Low	
Activity Level	☐ High	☐ Med	☐ Low	

FOOD INTAKE

Time	Food	Triggers/Reactions

A Holistic Approach to Eczema and Psoriasis

Self-Care Rituals: Make time for self-care rituals that promote relaxation and well-being.

NOTES

Date: ___/___/___

_____
_____
_____
_____

MOOD

☐ Hopeful ☐ Angry ☐ Bored

☐ Inspired ☐ Anxious ☐ Tired

☐ Happy ☐ Sad ☐ _____

WATER INTAKE

U U U
U U U
U U U
U U U

				Weather
Sleep	☐ High	☐ Med	☐ Low	
Energy Level	☐ High	☐ Med	☐ Low	
Activity Level	☐ High	☐ Med	☐ Low	

FOOD INTAKE

Time	Food	Triggers/Reactions

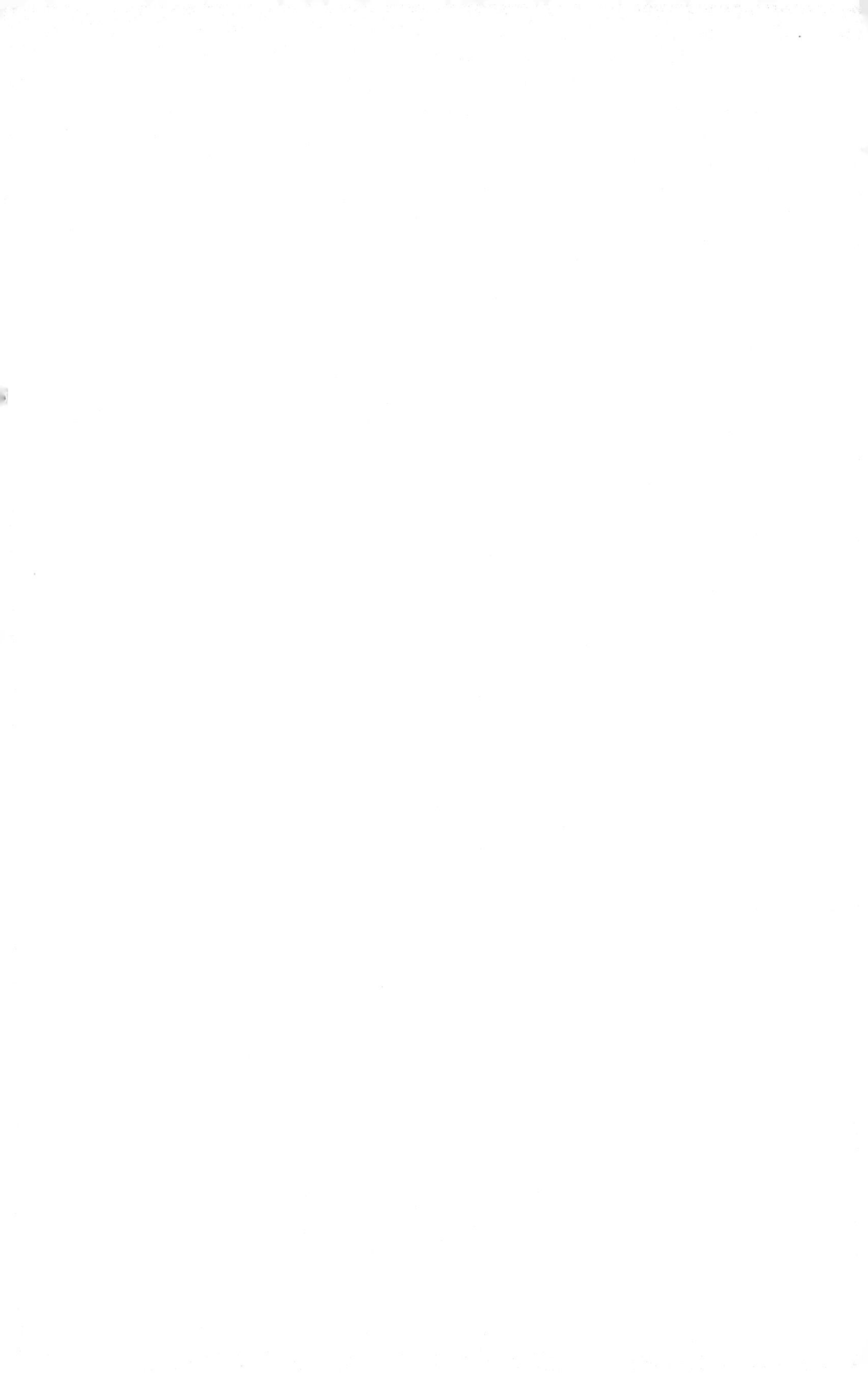

Printed in Great Britain
by Amazon